Central Pain Syndrome

A Beginner's Quick Start Guide to Managing CPS Through Diet and Other Natural Methods, With Sample Curated Recipes

mf

copyright © 2022 Patrick Marshwell

All rights reserved No part of this book may be reproduced, or stored in a retrieval system, or transmitted in any form or by any means, electronic, mechanical, photocopying, recording, or otherwise, without express written permission of the publisher.

Disclaimer

By reading this disclaimer, you are accepting the terms of the disclaimer in full. If you disagree with this disclaimer, please do not read the guide.

All of the content within this guide is provided for informational and educational purposes only, and should not be accepted as independent medical or other professional advice. The author is not a doctor, physician, nurse, mental health provider, or registered nutritionist/dietician. Therefore, using and reading this guide does not establish any form of a physician-patient relationship.

Always consult with a physician or another qualified health provider with any issues or questions you might have regarding any sort of medical condition. Do not ever disregard any qualified professional medical advice or delay seeking that advice because of anything you have read in this guide. The information in this guide is not intended to be any sort of medical advice and should not be used in lieu of any medical advice by a licensed and qualified medical professional.

The information in this guide has been compiled from a variety of known sources. However, the author cannot attest to or guarantee the accuracy of each source and thus should not be held liable for any errors or omissions.

You acknowledge that the publisher of this guide will not be held liable for any loss or damage of any kind incurred as a result of this guide or the reliance on any information provided within this guide. You acknowledge and agree that you assume all risk and responsibility for any action you undertake in response to the information in this guide.

Using this guide does not guarantee any particular result (e.g., weight loss or a cure). By reading this guide, you acknowledge that there are no guarantees to any specific outcome or results you can expect.

All product names, diet plans, or names used in this guide are for identification purposes only and are the property of their respective owners. The use of these names does not imply endorsement. All other trademarks cited herein are the property of their respective owners.

Where applicable, this guide is not intended to be a substitute for the original work of this diet plan and is, at most, a supplement to the original work for this diet plan and never a direct substitute. This guide is a personal expression of the facts of that diet plan.

Where applicable, persons shown in the cover images are stock photography models and the publisher has obtained the rights to use the images through license agreements with third-party stock image companies.

Table of Contents

Introduction	**7**
What Causes Central Pain Syndrome?	**9**
What Are the Symptoms of Central Pain Syndrome?	**13**
How Is CPS Diagnosed?	**16**
What Are the Medical Treatments for Central Pain Syndrome? 19	
How to Prevent Central Pain Syndrome?	**22**
How to manage CPS through natural methods?	23
Managing Central Pain Syndrome Through Diet and Nutrition 26	
Sample Recipes	**28**
Arugula and Mushroom Salad	29
Asparagus and Greens Salad with Tahini and Poppy Seed Dressing	30
Cauliflower Rice	31
Roasted Pumpkin and Brussel Sprouts	32
Apple in Pork Chops	33
Cauliflower Rice with Chicken and Broccoli	35
Chicken Stir Fry	36
Ginger Chicken Stir Fry	38
Roasted Chicken Thighs	40
Chicken Enchiladas	41
Cheddar Turkey Deviled Egg	43
Low FODMAP Burger	45
Steak with Mushroom Stroganoff	46
Lifestyle Changes to Manage Central Pain Syndrome	**48**
Exercise	48
Stress Management	49
Long-Term Outlook for People With CPS	50
Conclusion	**51**

FAQ About Central Pain Syndrome 52
References and Helpful Links 54

Introduction

Central pain syndrome is a neurological condition caused by damage to or dysfunction of the central nervous system (CNS), which includes the brain, brainstem, and spinal cord. This can result from a variety of injuries or diseases, such as stroke, multiple sclerosis, spinal cord injury, and cerebral palsy.

Symptoms vary depending on the person and the extent of the damage to the CNS but can include burning or aching pain, hypersensitivity to touch or temperature changes, muscle spasms, fatigue, and problems with coordination and balance. There is no cure for central pain syndrome, but there are treatments that can help lessen the symptoms.

Furthermore, it is important to note that central pain syndrome is a chronic condition, which means that it can last for months or years. It is important to seek medical help if you think you or a loved one may be experiencing any of the above symptoms.

In this quick start guide, we'll talk about:

- What causes central pain syndrome?
- What are the symptoms of central pain syndrome?
- How is central pain syndrome diagnosed?
- What are the medical treatments for central pain syndrome?
- How to prevent central pain syndrome?
- How to manage central pain syndrome through natural methods?
- Managing central pain syndrome through diet.

So, without further ado, let's get started with central pain syndrome.

What Causes Central Pain Syndrome?

Central pain syndrome (CPS) is a condition characterized by chronic pain that occurs in the central nervous system. The cause of CPS is unknown, but it is believed to be the result of damage to or dysfunction of the central nervous system. This can occur as a result of injury, disease, or surgery.

Specifically, CPS has been associated with the following:

Stroke

One of the most common causes of CPS is stroke. While the cause of CPS is still not fully understood, researchers believe that stroke may play a role in its development. Studies have shown that people who have had a stroke are more likely to develop CPS than those who have not had a stroke. Strokes can damage the parts of the brain that control movement and balance, which may lead to the development of CPS.

In addition, stroke can also cause inflammation and scarring in the brain, which may also contribute to the development of CPS. More research is needed to confirm the role of stroke in the development of CPS, but it is clear that stroke is a significant risk factor for this condition.

Multiple sclerosis

Multiple sclerosis (MS) is an autoimmune disease that attacks the central nervous system. It is one of the most common causes of Central Pain Syndrome. MS typically manifests as episodes of focal neurologic deficits that develop over days to weeks and remit partially or completely, with or without treatment.

The cause of MS is unknown, but it is thought to be an autoimmune disorder in which the body's immune system attacks myelin, the fatty substance that surrounds and protects nerve fibers in the central nervous system.

This damage disrupts communication between the brain and the body and can lead to a wide range of symptoms, including muscle weakness, paralysis, loss of sensation, problems with vision and balance, and cognitive impairment.

Spinal cord injury

Spinal cord injury (SCI) is another leading cause of central pain syndrome. The most common SCIs are due to car accidents, falls, and sports injuries. These injuries can damage the spinal cord and the nerves that run through it, causing pain signals to be sent to the brain even when there is no injury or damage. In some cases, SCI can also lead to inflammation and nerve damage.

Cerebral palsy

Cerebral palsy (CP) is one condition that has been linked to CPS. CP is a neurological disorder that affects movement and muscle tone. It is caused by damage to the brain, typically during early development. Studies have found that people with CP are more likely to experience CPS than those without CP. However, it is important to note that not all people with CP will develop CPS.

Other causes

Central pain syndrome can be brought on by a wide range of illnesses; however, brain tumors, epilepsy, Alzheimer's disease, and Parkinson's disease are among the less common causes of this disorder.

In cases where central pain syndrome is caused by a brain tumor, the tumor itself is not usually the source of the pain. However, the pressure that the tumor puts on nearby structures can cause pain.

In cases of epilepsy, central pain syndrome may be caused by damage to the thalamus, which is a key part of the brain's pain-processing system.

Central pain syndrome is a symptom that can be brought on by several neurodegenerative conditions, including Parkinson's disease and Alzheimer's disease.

- In Alzheimer's disease, central pain syndrome may be caused by damage to the hippocampus, which is involved in memory and learning.
- In Parkinson's disease, central pain syndrome may be caused by damage to the substantia nigra, which is involved in movement control.

Even though these are some of the less common causes of central pain syndrome, it is essential to bear in mind that any ailment that results in damage to the nervous system has the potential to lead to central pain syndrome.

Although the precise etiology of CPS is still a mystery, it is hoped that more investigation may assist in explaining this complex illness.

What Are the Symptoms of Central Pain Syndrome?

The symptoms of CPS vary depending on the person and the extent of damage to the CNS. However, common symptoms include:

Burning or aching pain

One symptom of central pain syndrome is burning or aching pain. This type of pain is often described as feeling like a hot poker is being pressed against the skin or like a severe sunburn. The pain can be constant or intermittent, and it may worsen with movement. It is often worse at night, making it difficult to sleep. The intensity of the pain can vary from mild to debilitating. In some cases, the pain may be accompanied by sensitivity to touch or temperature changes.

Hypersensitivity to touch or temperature changes

People with CPS often find that light touch, such as from clothing or a gentle breeze, is unbearable. They may also have difficulty regulating their body temperature, feeling too hot or too cold even when the room temperature hasn't changed. This can make everyday activities, such as taking a shower or getting dressed, extremely painful. In some cases, people with CPS become so sensitive to touch and temperature changes that they become isolated and unable to participate in the activities they once enjoyed.

Muscle spasms

One of the most common symptoms of central pain syndrome is muscle spasms. Muscle spasms are involuntary contractions of the muscles that can be painful and often disruptive. They can occur in any muscle group but are most common in the legs and arms. In some cases, they can be so severe that they interfere with daily activities. Muscle spasms are often treated with medication, physical therapy, and massage.

Fatigue

One of the most common symptoms of central pain syndrome (CPS) is fatigue. This fatigue can be both physical and mental, and it can have a significant impact on a person's quality of life. The exact cause of CPS-related fatigue is not known, but it is thought to be associated with changes in the way the brain processes pain signals.

Problems with coordination and balance

One symptom of central pain syndrome is problems with coordination and balance. Patients may find it difficult to walk or stand and may suffer from frequent falls. Coordination problems can also make it difficult to perform everyday tasks, such as dressing or bathing.

In addition, patients may experience a loss of sensation in their extremities, which can make it difficult to know where their limbs are in space. As a result, many patients with central pain syndrome require assistance with activities of daily living. Although there is no cure for central pain syndrome, treatments are available that can help to improve the quality of life.

Other problems such as anxiety, depression, and sleeping disorders

CPS can also lead to other problems such as anxiety, depression, and sleeping disorders. In some cases, the pain of CPS can be so severe that it leads to suicidal thoughts or attempts. If you are experiencing any of these symptoms, it is important to seek medical help. While there is no cure for CPS, there are treatments that can help to improve the quality of life for those who suffer from the condition.

The symptoms of CPS can vary in severity. Some people experience only mild symptoms, while others may be severely disabled. There is no cure for CPS, but there are treatments that can help lessen the symptoms.

How Is CPS Diagnosed?

Because CPS so frequently occurs in conjunction with other diseases, such as fibromyalgia or migraine headaches, it can be challenging to make a diagnosis of the disorder.

No one test can diagnose central pain syndrome. Instead, your physician will most likely employ a combination of the following treatments:

Medical history

Your medical history, including past injuries and illnesses, will be examined by your attending physician at some point. Additionally, he or she will inquire about the health of your family members. Your physician will also inquire about the onset of your symptoms and when they first appeared. They are going to be interested in finding out what makes your discomfort better or worse.

Physical exam

Your doctor will conduct a physical assessment on you to search for signs of complex regional pain syndrome (CRPS), such as allodynia (pain in reaction to a stimulus that does not ordinarily trigger pain) and hyperalgesia (increased pain in response to a stimulus that would normally cause pain).

Imaging tests

Imaging tests may be ordered by a doctor in addition to performing a physical exam on a patient and gathering the patient's medical history to rule out the possibility of other disorders that can cause similar symptoms.

Magnetic resonance imaging (MRI) and computed tomography (CT) scans are two of the most used tests because of their ability to offer detailed images of the brain and spinal cord. In certain cases, the symptoms of central pain syndrome might be confused with those of other disorders, such as stroke or multiple sclerosis. These photos can help determine whether or not these other conditions are present.

Neurological exam

Depending on what is thought to be the root of the problem, a neurological examination may be conducted to look for signs of central pain syndrome. In most cases, it includes an assessment of the patient's strength, sensitivity, and deep tendon reflexes, as well as coordination. The examiner might also evaluate the patient's mental status, level of consciousness, and the function of their cranial nerves.

Laboratory tests

Your doctor may order blood tests or other laboratory tests to rule out other conditions.

What Are the Medical Treatments for Central Pain Syndrome?

However, some therapies can help minimize the symptoms of central pain syndrome, even if there is no cure for the condition. These are the following:

Medications

Treatment for central pain syndrome often includes medications such as:

- Tricyclic antidepressants are commonly used to help relieve pain. They work by inhibiting the reuptake of neurotransmitters, which helps to reduce pain signals.
- Anticonvulsants are also commonly used to treat central pain syndrome. They work by reducing the excitability of neurons and preventing seizures.
- Painkillers are also often prescribed to help relieve pain. They work by blocking the pain signal from the nervous system.

Physical therapy

There is currently no known cure for CPS; however, there are therapies available that may help alleviate some of the symptoms. One example of such a treatment is physical therapy. Patients suffering from CPS can benefit from the assistance of physical therapists in improving their range of motion and experiencing less discomfort.

In addition to this, physical therapy can also be of use in preventing more injury to the neurological system. As a consequence of this, patients diagnosed with CPS should incorporate physical therapy into their overall treatment strategy.

Occupational therapy

Occupational therapy has the potential to be an effective treatment for complex regional pain syndrome. Occupational therapists are trained to help patients learn how to alter their everyday routines and activities to accommodate their medical conditions. They are also able to supply you with the instruments and methods that can assist you in managing your discomfort. If you have CPS, you should discuss the possibility of participating in occupational therapy with your primary care provider.

Surgery

Surgery may be the most effective course of treatment for central pain syndrome in certain instances. It is not suggested in most cases unless there is an underlying ailment that is causing the pain and when other treatment options have been tried and found to be ineffective. It is possible to repair damage to the nervous system by surgery, as well as remove tumors or other growths that are putting pressure on nerves.

Additionally, it can be utilized to ease the pressure that is being placed on the spinal cord. It is vital to keep in mind that even while surgery helps alleviate pain in the majority of cases, there is always a danger of consequences.

Before settling on a choice, anyone who is thinking about undergoing surgical procedures ought to discuss with their primary care physician about the potential downsides and upsides of the procedure.

How to Prevent Central Pain Syndrome?

There is no sure way to prevent central pain syndrome, but there are some things you can do to lower your risk. These include:

Managing conditions that can lead to central pain syndrome: Central pain syndrome is a condition that can be caused by a variety of underlying conditions, including stroke, trauma, and disease. While there is no cure for central pain syndrome, there are ways to manage the condition and help prevent it from developing.

One of the most important things you can do is to manage any underlying conditions you may have. This may involve taking medications, exercising, and eating a healthy diet. By keeping your condition under control, you can help to reduce your risk of developing central pain syndrome.

In addition, it's important to be aware of the signs and symptoms of central pain syndrome so that you can seek treatment as soon as possible if you do develop the condition.

With proper management, central pain syndrome can be effectively managed and its impact on your life minimized.

Avoiding injuries

Injuries to the central nervous system are one of the potential triggers for central pain syndrome. Central pain syndrome can be brought on by a variety of conditions, including spinal cord injuries, brain injuries, strokes, and multiple sclerosis. Spinal cord injuries are the most common cause of this condition.

The greatest method for preventing central pain syndrome is to avoid getting injured in the first place, as this is one of the potential causes of the disorder. When engaging in activities that come with a high probability of injury, taking precautions like donning protective clothing and equipment can help cut down on the likelihood of acquiring central pain syndrome.

How to manage CPS through natural methods?

You can find relief from your symptoms with the help of several different natural remedies. The following are some of these:

Diet

One approach to managing CPS is through diet. A healthy diet can help to reduce inflammation and pain, and it can also provide the nutrients needed for healing. Some nutrient-rich foods that may help to ease CPS symptoms include omega-3 fatty acids, magnesium, vitamin B6, and Boswellia. In addition to eating a healthy diet, it is also important to stay hydrated. Drinking plenty of water helps to flush toxins from the body and can help reduce pain and inflammation.

Exercise

Additionally, regular exercise is an effective treatment for CPS. It has been proven that regular exercise can improve the function of the central nervous system and lower the amount of pain experienced by persons who suffer from CPS. In addition, physical activity has been shown to assist improve mood as well as the quality of sleep, both of which are frequently disrupted in persons who have CPS. As a consequence of this, physical activity has the potential to be an advantageous supplement to the therapy of CPS.

Stress management

Stress management is a key component of managing central pain syndrome. When the body is under stress, it releases hormones that can aggravate the pain symptoms associated with central pain syndrome. As a result, it is important to find ways to manage stress to minimize its impact on the body. This may include relaxation techniques, such as yoga or meditation.

Acupuncture

Though often overlooked, acupuncture is a key natural method that can be used to help manage central pain syndrome. By stimulating points in the body, acupuncture can help to release endorphins and other neurotransmitters that can help to block pain signals. In addition, acupuncture can help to increase blood flow and reduce inflammation.

As a result, this centuries-old practice can be an effective way to address the chronic pain associated with central pain syndrome. Though it is not a cure, acupuncture can provide significant relief and improve the quality of life for those struggling with this condition.

Massage

Massage therapy can help reduce pain, improve the range of motion, and increase circulation. In addition, massage can help to reduce stress and promote relaxation. For people with CPS, massage may provide significant relief from chronic pain and help them to better manage their condition.

Managing Central Pain Syndrome Through Diet and Nutrition

What you eat can have a big impact on your symptoms. Eating a healthy diet that includes plenty of fruits, vegetables, and whole grains can help reduce inflammation and pain. You may also want to avoid processed foods, sugar, and caffeine. In addition, staying hydrated by drinking plenty of water is important.

Here are some specific dietary recommendations to help you manage central pain syndrome:

Increase your intake of anti-inflammatory foods

Anti-inflammatory foods include omega-3 fatty acids, turmeric, ginger, and green leafy vegetables. Adding these to your diet can help reduce inflammation and pain.

Get enough protein

Protein is important for repairing the tissues in your body. Therefore, getting enough protein is essential for managing central pain syndrome. Good sources of protein include chicken, fish, tofu, beans, and lentils.

Increase your intake of vitamins and minerals

Vitamins and minerals are important for maintaining your health. Some specific vitamins and minerals that can help reduce pain include vitamin D, magnesium, and calcium.

Avoid trigger foods

Some people find that certain foods trigger their symptoms. Common trigger foods include nightshade vegetables, such as tomatoes and potatoes, and gluten. If you suspect that a certain food is triggering your symptoms, try eliminating it from your diet to see if your symptoms improve.

Sample Recipes

Arugula and Mushroom Salad

Ingredients:

- 5 oz. arugula washed
- 1 lb. fresh mushrooms
- 1/4 tsp. shoyu
- 1/2 red onion
- 1 tbsp. olive oil
- 1 tbsp. mirin

For tofu cheese:

- • 1/8 cup umeboshi vinegar
- • 1/2 firm tofu

Instructions:

1. In a bowl, add the rinsed tofu. Crumble and pour in vinegar.
2. In a separate bowl add shoyu, red onions, salt, olive oil, and mirin. 3. Mix to combine.
3. Add in the arugula and toss to combine with the dressing.
4. Serve and enjoy.

Asparagus and Greens Salad with Tahini and Poppy Seed Dressing

Ingredients:

- 10 to 12 asparagus stalks, washed well and sliced into ribbons
- 5 radishes, washed well and sliced thinly
- 2 to 3 rainbow carrots, peeled and sliced thinly
- 1 handful wild spinach
- 1 small handful of microgreens, washed well
- 1 small handful of sunflower greens, washed well
- optional: few pieces of chive blossoms

For the dressing:

- 2 tbsp. tahini
- 1 tbsp. poppy seeds
- 1 tbsp. extra-virgin olive oil
- salt
- pepper

Instructions:

1. For the dressing, whisk ingredients together in a small bowl.
2. In a separate bowl, toss salad ingredients into the mixture.
3. Drizzle dressing on salad upon serving.

Cauliflower Rice

Ingredients:

- 1 head cauliflower, coarsely grated for grainy texture
- 1 tbsp. organic coconut oil
- 1/2 cup yellow onion, chopped
- 1 tsp. Primal Palate garlic and herb seasoning
- 1 clove garlic, minced
- 1/2 tsp. Himalayan pink salt, to taste

Instructions:

1. Put a skillet on medium heat. Add coconut oil.
2. Put in the onion and garlic and sauté for 3 to 4 minutes.
3. Add the cauliflower grains and continue to sauté the mixture for another 4 to 5 minutes.
4. Flavor the cauliflower rice with salt before serving.
5. Serve while warm.

Roasted Pumpkin and Brussel Sprouts

Ingredients:

- 3 lb. pie pumpkin, peeled and cut into ¾-inch cubes
- 1 lb. fresh Brussels sprouts, trimmed and halved lengthwise
- 1 tsp. sea salt
- 1/2 tsp. coarsely ground pepper
- 1/3 cup olive oil
- 2 tbsp. balsamic vinegar
- 2 tbsp. minced fresh parsley
- 4 garlic cloves, thinly sliced

Instructions:

1. Preheat the oven to 400°F.
2. Combine Brussels sprouts, garlic, and pumpkin in a bowl.
3. Whisk oil, vinegar, salt, and pepper in a separate bowl.
4. Drizzle the mixture over the vegetables. Toss gently.
5. Pour the coated vegetables onto a greased baking pan.
6. until tender, about 35-40 minutes. Stir once.
7. Sprinkle with parsley upon serving.

Apple in Pork Chops

Ingredients:

- 1 tbsp. onion, chopped
- 1/4 cup celery, chopped
- 2 cups apples, chopped
- 2 tsp. fresh parsley, chopped
- 3 cups bread crumbs, fresh
- 6 pcs. thick pork chops, 1.25"
- 1 tbsp. vegetable oil
- 1/4 cup butter
- 1/4 tsp. + more salt
- pepper

Instructions:

1. Preheat the oven to 350°F.
2. Heat butter in a large skillet, and saute onion. Remove from heat.
3. Mix in apples, bread crumbs, celery, parsley, and 1/4 teaspoon salt. Set aside the apple mixture
4. Cut open a side of the pork chop to create a pocket.
5. Season it with salt and pepper, both in the pocket and the entire pork chop.
6. Add a spoonful of apple mixture into the pockets. Don't stuff it in.
7. Heat up oil in a skillet over medium-high heat. Cook chops until both sides are brown.

8. Transfer to a 9x13-inch baking dish that is ungreased. Cover with aluminum foil.
9. Bake in the oven for half an hour.
10. Remove the foil and bake for another half hour or until the juices look clear.

Cauliflower Rice with Chicken and Broccoli

Ingredients:

- 1 broccoli head
- 1 cauliflower head
- 2 chicken breasts, boneless and skinless
- 1 tbsp. olive oil
- salt
- pepper

Instructions:

1. Preheat the oven to 350°F.
2. Cut the broccoli into small florets.
3. Remove the core from the cauliflower and chop it into small pieces.
4. In a food processor, pulse the cauliflower until it resembles rice.
5. In a baking dish, combine broccoli, cauliflower rice, chicken, and olive oil. Season with salt and pepper.
6. Bake for 20-25 minutes, or until the chicken is cooked through.

This recipe features chicken, broccoli, and cauliflower rice, all of which are good protein sources. The broccoli provides calcium and vitamin K while the cauliflower rice is a low-carbohydrate alternative to traditional rice.

Chicken Stir Fry

Ingredients:

- 1 tbsp. coconut oil
- 2 chicken breasts, cubed
- 1 red bell pepper, diced
- 1 cup broccoli florets
- 1 large sweet potato, shredded or spiralized
- 2 tbsp. parsley, chopped
- 1 tbsp. sesame seeds
- 1 lime, wedged

For the Turmeric Sauce:

- 1/2 can coconut milk
- 1 tbsp. almond butter
- 2 cloves garlic, minced
- 1 lime juiced
- 1 tsp. turmeric
- 1 tsp. sea salt
- 1/2 tsp. ginger powder, add more to taste
- 1/2 tsp. pepper

Instructions:

1. In a large skillet or wok placed on medium-high heat, pour in the coconut oil.
2. Add chicken breasts and cook for 3-4 minutes per side

3. Add bell pepper, broccoli, and sweet potato noodles. Stir for 2-3 minutes.
4. While the chicken is cooking, whisk together the ingredients for the sauce.
5. Toss the mix with your spoon or tongs for 2-3 minutes.
6. Taste and adjust seasonings to your liking.
7. Top with parsley and sesame seeds.
8. Serve with lime wedges.

Ginger Chicken Stir Fry

Ingredients:

Stir-fry mix:

- 1 lb. cooked chicken, dark or light meat
- 4 cups cremini mushrooms, sliced
- 4 cups purple cabbage, sliced
- 2 cups carrots
- 1/2 cup green onions, cut slanted
- 3 cups cauliflower florets
- 1 handful enoki mushrooms
- 2 tbsp. avocado oil
- 1 package rice noodles, cook according to instructions

Stir-fry sauce:

- 4 cloves minced garlic
- 1/4 cup honey
- 1/4 tsp. grated ginger
- 1/4 cup rice wine vinegar
- 1 cup chicken stock
- 1 tbsp. avocado oil

Instructions:

To make the stir-fry sauce:

1. Cook garlic with oil on low to medium heat

2. Once the garlic is browned, add in the honey. Let the sauce bubble for a moment.
3. Add in the vinegar and cover with a lid.
4. Pour in the chicken stock. Leave to boil until reduced by half.
5. Season with salt and pepper.

To make the stir-fry mix:

1. Heat the oil in a large wok. Cook the vegetables, adding one-by-one according to the degree of hardness.
2. Once the vegetables are well-caramelized, add in the chicken and noodles and heat through.
3. Pour in the stir-fry sauce and mix well.
4. Garnish with green onions

Roasted Chicken Thighs

Ingredients:

- 12 garlic cloves, unpeeled
- 1 tbsp. avocado oil
- 1 pinch Himalayan pink salt
- 4 chicken thighs with skin
- 1 tsp. Primal Palate super gyro seasoning

Instructions:

1. Pour avocado oil over a medium-sized oven-safe pot.
2. Add the garlic cloves. Sauté over medium heat for 2 to 3 minutes or until the skins begin to brown.
3. Place the chicken in a large skillet over medium-high heat. Sear for about 2 to 3 minutes for each side, starting with the skin side.
4. Combine the chicken with the garlic. Season generously with salt and Primal Palate Super Gyro seasoning.
5. Place the chicken in an oven preheated to 350°F.
6. Bake for one hour while covered.
7. Serve and enjoy.

Chicken Enchiladas

Ingredients:

- 2 chicken breasts, skinless and boneless
- juice of 1 lime or 3 tbsp. bottled lime juice
- 1 tsp. dried garlic
- chimichurri sauce, or 1 bunch of cilantro pureed with 1 tbsp. olive oil
- 16 oz. package of sliced chicken or turkey sandwich meat
- 8 oz. spinach, cooked
- 8 oz. shredded cheese
- 1 bell pepper, sliced
- 1 jar of salsa verde or enchilada sauce

Instructions:

1. Place the chicken breasts in a crockpot and drizzle them with lime juice.
2. Pour chimichurri sauce or cilantro sauce.
3. Add in garlic.
4. Cook the chicken for 8 hours on low, or for 4-5 hours if set on high.
5. Remove cooked chicken from the crockpot.
6. Shred the chicken with two forks.

To make enchiladas:

1. Preheat the oven to 400°F.

2. Use 4 slices of the packaged meat to make the enchilada wrapper. Place 2 slices next to each other, slightly overlapping. Add 2 more, also overlapping slightly.
3. In the middle of the meat wrapper, create a small row of shredded chicken.
4. Add another row of each of the ingredients on one side, particularly the closest to you—spinach, strips of pepper strips, and half of the cheese.
5. Roll the enchilada by pulling the wrapper over the top of the filling. Carefully squeeze the filling to one side.
6. Keep rolling and squeezing, making sure that the fillings are wrapped tightly. Remember that the meat wrapper is not as firm as a regular flour-based tortilla wrapper.
7. Place the wrapped chicken in a pan with the seam side down.
8. Repeat until the enchiladas are in pan
9. Pour over two tbsp. of salsa verde or enchilada sauce.
10. Sprinkle the remaining cheese.
11. Place in the oven and bake for 12 to 15 minutes, or until the cheese is melted.
12. Serve and enjoy while warm.

Cheddar Turkey Deviled Egg

Ingredients:

- 6 large organic eggs
- 2 slices nitrate-free turkey bacon
- 1/4 cup low-fat cheddar cheese, shredded OR grated
- 3 tbsp. light mayonnaise
- 1 tsp. white wine vinegar
- 1/2 tsp. chives, chopped
- 1/8 tsp. ground black pepper
- 1/8 tsp. salt

Instructions:

1. Place the eggs in a large pot or saucepan.
2. Pour cold water into the pot or pan until the water is covering the eggs by 1-1/2 inches.
3. Bring the water to a boil over high heat.
4. Once it has boiled, remove it from the stove.
5. Cover and let it stand for 12 to 15 minutes.
6. When it has cooled down, peel off the egg's shells.
7. Fry the bacon slices using medium-high heat in a non-stick skillet until bacon slices have become crispy but not burnt.
8. Transfer fried bacon to paper towels to drain off the excess oil.
9. Once it has cooled down, break down the bacon into small bits. Set aside.

10. Cut the hard-boiled eggs into half, lengthwise.
11. Gently carve out the egg yolks into a medium-sized bowl.
12. Arrange the hollowed-out egg halves in a flat container.
13. Add the rest of the ingredients to the bowl with the yolk.
14. Stir well until the texture has become smooth.
15. Transfer the mixture into a piping bag or resealable bag with a trimmed corner.
16. Pipe the yolk mixture back into the egg halves.
17. Sprinkle each filled egg half with bacon bits.
18. Serve immediately or after it has been chilled for at least half an hour.

Low FODMAP Burger

Ingredients:

- 1-1/4 lbs. ground pork
- 1/4 tsp. allspice
- 1/2 tsp. salt
- 1/2 tsp. white pepper
- 1/2 tsp. ground nutmeg
- 1/2 tsp. caraway seeds
- 1/2 tsp. ground ginger

Instructions:

1. Preheat the grill then prepare the patty.
2. Using a small mixing bowl, stir together the salt, pepper, allspice, nutmeg, and ginger until fully combined.
3. Place the ground in a large mixing bowl and add the spice mixture.
4. Mix thoroughly until spices are evenly distributed to the pork.
5. Make round, flat burger patties using the palm of your hands.
6. Grill the patties and serve with gluten-free buns and mustard sauce.

Steak with Mushroom Stroganoff

Ingredients:

- 4 oz. rib-eye steak
- 3 tbsps. extra-virgin olive oil
- salt and pepper
- 4 oz. whole mushrooms, quartered
- 1 large clove garlic, minced
- 1 tsp. fresh parsley, minced
- 3 tbsps. chicken stock, or as needed
- 1-1/2 oz. hard cheese
- 1/4 tsp. black pepper, for the sauce
- 1/4 tsp Worcestershire sauce

Instructions:

1. Using a skillet, heat half of the olive oil over medium-high heat.
2. Sprinkle a pinch of salt and pepper over the steak then sear for 3-5 minutes. Set aside.
3. Using another pan, heat the rest of the olive oil and add the mushroom. Cook the mushroom until softened.
4. Lower the heat then add the garlic. Cook again for 12-2 minutes. Add the chicken stock and stir.
5. Add the Worcestershire sauce, hard cheese, and pepper. Blend the mixture well until the cheese incorporates into the sauce.

6. Serve the steak then add the finished mushroom stroganoff mixture. Garnish with parsley for presentation.

Lifestyle Changes to Manage Central Pain Syndrome

Exercise

Exercise is important for managing central pain syndrome. It can help improve your range of motion, reduce pain, and increase endorphins. However, it's important to talk to your doctor before starting an exercise program. This is because some exercises may worsen your symptoms.

Some exercises that may be helpful include:

Swimming

Swimming is a great exercise for people with central pain syndrome. It's low impact and can help improve your range of motion.

Yoga

Yoga can help improve your flexibility, reduce pain, and increase endorphins.

Tai chi

Tai chi is a form of martial arts that involves slow, graceful movements. It can help improve balance, flexibility, and pain.

Strength training

Strength-training exercises can help build muscle and reduce pain.

When starting an exercise program, it's important to start slow and gradually increase the intensity of your workouts. It's also important to listen to your body and stop if you're in pain.

Stress Management

Stress can worsen symptoms of central pain syndrome. Therefore, it's important to find ways to manage stress. This may include:

Relaxation techniques

Relaxation techniques such as yoga and meditation are often recommended for people with central pain syndrome. These activities can help to reduce stress and promote relaxation, which can in turn help to ease the symptoms of central pain syndrome.

Talking to a counselor or therapist

Talking to a counselor or therapist can help you learn how to deal with stress. They can also teach you coping mechanisms and provide support.

Long-Term Outlook for People With CPS

The long-term outlook for people with central pain syndrome varies. Some people may only have mild symptoms that can be managed with treatment. Others may have more severe symptoms that significantly affect their quality of life. There is currently no cure for central pain syndrome, but treatments can help lessen the symptoms.

If you or someone you know has central pain syndrome, there are many ways to get help and support. Talk to your doctor about treatment options and consider joining a support group. With proper treatment and self-care, it's possible to manage central pain syndrome and enjoy a good quality of life.

Conclusion

Central pain syndrome is a condition that causes pain. It can be caused by damage to the nervous system. There is no cure for central pain syndrome, but treatments can help lessen the symptoms. These include exercise, an anti-inflammatory diet, stress management, and alternative treatments. The long-term outlook for people with central pain syndrome varies.

Some people may only have mild symptoms while others may have more severe symptoms that significantly affect their quality of life. With proper treatment and self-care, it's possible to manage central pain syndrome and enjoy a good quality of life.

This quick start guide has provided you with an overview of central pain syndrome and some potential methods to manage this condition. If you or someone you know has central pain syndrome, talk to your doctor about treatment options. There are many ways to get help and support. With proper treatment and self-care, it's possible to manage central pain syndrome and enjoy a good quality of life.

FAQ About Central Pain Syndrome

Q: What is central pain syndrome?

A: Central pain syndrome is a condition that causes pain. It can be caused by damage to the nervous system.

Q: What are the symptoms of central pain syndrome?

A: Symptoms of central pain syndrome can vary. They may include pain, numbness, tingling, and muscle weakness.

Q: What causes central pain syndrome?

A: Central pain syndrome can be caused by damage to the nervous system. This may be due to an injury, surgery, stroke, or another condition.

Q: How is central pain syndrome diagnosed?

A: Central pain syndrome is typically diagnosed based on a person's symptoms and medical history. A physical exam may also be done.

Q: How is central pain syndrome treated?

A: There is no cure for central pain syndrome, but treatments can help lessen the symptoms. These include exercise, an anti-inflammatory diet, stress management, and alternative treatments.

Q: What is the long-term outlook for people with central pain syndrome?

A: The long-term outlook for people with central pain syndrome varies. Some people may only have mild symptoms while others may have more severe symptoms that significantly affect their quality of life. With proper treatment and self-care, it's possible to manage central pain syndrome and enjoy a good quality of life.

Q: What are some potential methods to manage central pain syndrome?

A: Potential methods to manage central pain syndrome include exercise, an anti-inflammatory diet, stress management, and alternative treatments. Talk to your doctor about which treatment options are best for you.

References and Helpful Links

Central Pain Syndrome (CPS): Medications, Definition, And More. (2014, December 1). Healthline. https://www.healthline.com/health/pain-relief-central-pain-syndrome.

Central Pain Syndrome | National Institute of Neurological Disorders and Stroke. (n.d.). Retrieved October 9, 2022, from https://www.ninds.nih.gov/health-information/disorders/central-pain-syndrome.

Central Pain Syndrome. (n.d.). NORD (National Organization for Rare Disorders). Retrieved October 9, 2022, from https://rarediseases.org/rare-diseases/central-pain-syndrome/.

Yasaei, R., Peterson, E., & Saadabadi, A. (2022). Chronic pain syndrome. In StatPearls. StatPearls Publishing. http://www.ncbi.nlm.nih.gov/books/NBK470523/.

www.ingramcontent.com/pod-product-compliance
Lightning Source LLC
LaVergne TN
LVHW051924060526
838201LV00062B/4670